THE COMPLETE MEDITERRANEAN DIET COOKBOOK FOR CHRONIC KIDNEY DISEASE

Super Easy Flavorful and Vibrant Mediterranean Recipes to Manage Chronic Renal Disease.

DOROTHY R MILLER

Disclaimer Notice:

The information provided in this book is for general informational purposes only. The author and publisher are not liable for any damages or injuries resulting from the use of the content in this book. The reader assumes full responsibility for their actions and decisions based on the information herein.

The exercises, poses, and health tips mentioned in this book are intended for general audiences, including seniors, but individual results may vary. Before starting any new exercise or wellness program, it is advisable to consult with a qualified healthcare professional, especially for individuals with pre-existing health conditions or concerns.

The author and publisher have made every effort to ensure the accuracy and completeness of the information provided in this book. However, they do not guarantee the efficacy or suitability of the practices for every individual. Readers should use their discretion and judgment in applying the content to their specific circumstances.

By reading this book, the reader acknowledges and agrees to the terms of this disclaimer.

Dear Valued Reader,

Thank you for choosing **"The Complete Mediterranean Diet Cookbook for Chronic Kidney Disease"**! Your support means the world to me.

If you enjoyed the book and found it valuable, I would be immensely grateful if you could take a moment to leave a review. Your feedback not only helps other readers discover the book but also guides me in creating better content for you.

Your honest thoughts and opinions are highly appreciated. Please share your review.

Thank you once again for being a part of this journey!

Warm regards,

Gain access to my other exciting books on this QR CODE, Just scan it as simple as that.

Here is my email QR CODE

Feel free to send me email at

rmillerdorothy51@gmail.com

" If you have any question regarding this book, I will be at your service any day anytime, feedback within two hours."

I also offer free consultation anytime as a doctor via my email. Thank you for your purchase

TABLE OF CONTENT

CHAPTER ONE

INTRODUCTION

First of All, Welcome to the Complete Mediterranean Diet Cookbook for Chronic Kidney Disease.

Before we dive into this life changing journey let me tell you a moving and motivational story on how Mediterranean diet cookbook helps Robert heal chronic kidney disease (CKD).

In the heart of an adorable city nestled between rolling hills, lived an unassuming senior called Robert. Once a vibrant soul, his days had gradually darkened as the weight of chronic kidney disease began to cast its shadow over his life. Every step became an arduous trip, every meal a meticulous calculation. But Robert's spirit stayed unbroken.

Amidst the battle, a ray of hope emerged when Robert stumbled upon the virtues of the Mediterranean diet. Encouraged by the whispers of wellness, he went on a culinary adventure that would transform not just his meals but his entire life.

With unwavering determination, Robert accepted this new way of nourishing his body. The aroma of fresh herbs lingered in his kitchen as he carefully prepared colorful plates brimming with vibrant vegetables, succulent fish, and the golden hues of extra virgin olive oil. Each meal was a symphony of flavors, carefully created to heal from within.

As days turned into weeks, a miraculous change began to emerge. His energy, once stolen by tiredness, returned in joyful bursts. The heavy weight that had shackled him for so long began to lighten. A newfound glow danced upon his weathered face, bringing tales of renewal and hope.

But it wasn't just physical renewal that graced Robert's life. The newfound joy of savoring each bite, the thrill of exploring fresh produce at the market, and the warmth of sharing meals with newfound friends rejuvenated his soul. The Mediterranean diet became not just a routine but a way of life—a tapestry woven with love, laughter, and a celebration of each passing day.

Through the healing power of wholesome ingredients and mindful eating, Robert discovered not just a better lifestyle but a deep love for the simple joys of life. Surrounded by the embrace of newfound health and a heart brimming with thanks, he found himself living each day happily, savoring the rich flavors of existence once more.

Now you heard how Roberts fight with (CKD) and finally won, I brought this story up so that it will motivate you and for you to know that you can do it too.

Now let's start the journey together

Chronic Kidney Disease (CKD)

Chronic Kidney Disease refers to the gradual loss of kidney function over time. It's a long-term condition where the kidneys don't work effectively to filter waste and excess fluids from the blood.

Types Of CKD

1. **Stage Progression:** CKD is categorized into stages based on the level of kidney function, from Stage 1 (mild) to Stage 5 (kidney failure).

2. **Specific Causes:** CKD can be caused by diabetes, high blood pressure (hypertension), glomerulonephritis, polycystic kidney disease, urinary tract obstructions, and other conditions.

Causes Of CKD

1. **Diabetes:** High blood sugar levels over time can damage the kidneys.

2. **<u>High Blood Pressure:</u>** Prolonged high blood pressure can strain the kidneys.

3. **<u>Glomerulonephritis:</u>** Inflammation of the kidney's filtering units.

4. **<u>Other Health Issues:</u>** Kidney stones, urinary tract infections, prolonged obstruction in the urinary tract, and genetic diseases.

Symptoms Of CKD

1. **<u>Fatigue and Weakness:</u>** Due to anemia.

2. **<u>Swelling:</u>** Especially in the legs, ankles, or around the eyes.

3. **<u>Changes in Urination:</u>** Frequent urination, especially at night, blood in urine, foamy urine.

4. **<u>Shortness of Breath:</u>** Due to fluid buildup in the lungs.

5. **Nausea and Vomiting:** Caused by the accumulation of waste in the body.

Preventive Measures For CKD

1. **Manage Blood Sugar**: Control diabetes through medication, diet, and exercise.

2. **Manage Blood Pressure:** Regular check-ups and medication to control hypertension.

3. **Healthy Lifestyle:** Maintain a balanced diet, regular exercise, limit alcohol intake, avoid smoking.

4. **Regular Health Checks:** Monitor kidney function through routine check-ups and screenings, especially if you have risk factors or a family history of kidney disease.

Early detection and proper management of underlying conditions can significantly slow the progression of CKD and help maintain better kidney function.

CHAPTER TWO

BENEFITS OF MEDITERRANEAN DIET TO (CKD) PATIENTS

The Mediterranean diet has gained attention for its potential benefits in managing chronic kidney disease (CKD). Here's why it's considered important and how it helps:

1. **Nutrient Balance:** The Mediterranean diet emphasizes fresh fruits, vegetables, whole grains, lean proteins (like fish and poultry), and healthy fats (like olive oil and nuts). This balance provides essential nutrients without overloading the kidneys with excessive protein or sodium.

2. **Lower Sodium Intake:** It typically contains lower amounts of sodium compared to many Western diets. This can help

manage blood pressure, a crucial aspect in slowing the progression of CKD.

3. **<u>Healthy Fats:</u>** The diet includes monounsaturated fats from olive oil and omega-3 fatty acids from fish, which are heart-healthy and may benefit kidney health by reducing inflammation.

4. **<u>Reduced Red Meat:</u>** Reducing intake of red meat in favor of leaner protein sources helps lower the burden on the kidneys, as excess protein can strain kidney function.

5. **<u>Antioxidants and Anti-inflammatory Properties:</u>** The diet is rich in antioxidants and anti-inflammatory compounds from fruits, vegetables, and olive oil. These properties can help reduce inflammation and oxidative stress in the body, potentially benefiting kidney health.

6. **<u>Weight Management:</u>** The Mediterranean diet, when combined with regular exercise, can aid in weight

management. Maintaining a healthy weight is essential for managing CKD and reducing associated complications.

Remember, while diet plays a crucial role, it's part of a holistic approach to managing CKD. Medication adherence, lifestyle modifications, and regular monitoring by healthcare providers remain integral in controlling and slowing the progression of chronic kidney disease.

30-DAY SAMPLE MEAL PLAN FOR MEDITERRANEAN DIET FOR (CKD)

An easy-to-follow meal plan to start your journey

Day 1-3:

Breakfast: Greek yogurt with honey and berries.

Lunch: Grilled chicken or chickpea salad with mixed greens, tomatoes, cucumbers, olives, and feta cheese.

Dinner: Baked fish with roasted vegetables (like zucchini, bell peppers, and onions) and quinoa.

Snacks: Mixed nuts, carrot sticks with hummus.

Day 4-5:

Breakfast: Oatmeal with fresh fruit and nuts.

Lunch: Whole grain wrap with grilled vegetables, hummus, and a side salad.

Dinner: Pasta primavera with whole grain pasta, tossed with seasonal vegetables and olive oil.

Snacks: Greek yogurt with sliced almonds, apple slices.

Day 6-7:

Breakfast: Whole grain toast with avocado and a poached egg.

Lunch: Lentil soup with a side of whole grain bread and a Greek salad.

Dinner: Grilled salmon with a spinach and tomato salad.

Snacks: Fresh fruit, cheese with whole grain crackers.

Day 8-10:

Breakfast: Smoothie with spinach, banana, berries, and Greek yogurt.

Lunch: Quinoa tabbouleh with grilled chicken or tofu.

Dinner: Ratatouille (a mix of eggplant, zucchini, bell peppers, tomatoes) with a side of couscous.

Snacks: Hummus with whole grain pita, mixed nuts.

Day 11-12:

Breakfast: Frittata with spinach, tomatoes, and feta cheese.

Lunch: Whole grain wrap with grilled veggies and falafel.

Dinner: Chicken or vegetable paella with a side salad.

Snacks: Olives, carrot sticks with tzatziki.

Day 13-15:

Breakfast: Greek yogurt parfait with granola and fresh fruit.

Lunch: Whole grain pasta with pesto, cherry tomatoes, and grilled chicken or tofu.

Dinner: Grilled shrimp with quinoa and a side of roasted vegetables.

Snacks: Mixed nuts, apple slices with almond butter.

Continue alternating and mixing these meal ideas throughout the 30-day period, ensuring a variety of nutrients and flavors. Also, make sure to drink plenty of water and, if needed, consult with a nutritionist or healthcare professional for personalized guidance.

HOW TO FOLLOW THIS MEDITERRANEAN DIET

Sure, here are some guidelines to follow the Mediterranean diet effectively:

Emphasize on plant-based

1. **Vegetables & Fruits:** Aim for a variety of colorful veggies and fruits daily.

2. **Whole Grains:** Choose whole grain bread, pasta, couscous, and brown rice over refined grains.

3. **Legumes & Nuts:** Incorporate beans, lentils, chickpeas, and a variety of nuts and seeds.

Healthy Fats

1. **Olive Oil:** Use extra virgin olive oil as the primary source of fat.

2. **Fatty Fish:** Include fish like salmon, mackerel, and sardines for omega-3 fatty acids.

3. **Nuts & Seeds:** Snack on nuts and seeds like almonds, walnuts, and chia seeds.

Moderate Dairy & Poultry

1. **Dairy:** Greek yogurt and cheese in moderation.
2. **Poultry:** Chicken and turkey a few times a week, focusing more on fish.

Limit Red Meat & Processed Foods

1. **Red Meat:** Limit consumption of red meat to a few times a month.
2. **Processed Foods:** Minimize intake of processed foods and fast food.

Herbs & Spices for Flavor

1. **Seasonings:** Use herbs and spices for flavor instead of excessive salt.

2. **Garlic & Onions:** Incorporate these aromatic vegetables for added taste.

Enjoy Meals Mindfully

1. **Portion Control:** Pay attention to portion sizes, and avoid overeating.
2. **Slow Eating:** Chew food thoroughly and savor each bite mindfully.
3. **Social Meals:** Enjoy meals with family or friends whenever possible.

Hydration & Beverages

1. **Water:** Stay hydrated by drinking plenty of water throughout the day.
2. **Moderate Wine:** If desired, enjoy red wine in moderation (1 glass per day for women, 2 for men).

Physical Activity & Lifestyle

1. **Regular Exercise:** Combine the diet with regular physical activity for overall health benefits.

2. **Stress Management:** Incorporate stress-reducing activities like yoga or meditation.

Meal Planning and Preparation

1. **Plan Ahead:** Plan meals and snacks in advance to maintain consistency.

2. **Cook at Home:** Prepare meals at home using fresh, whole ingredients.

Following these guidelines while incorporating the suggested meal plans can help you adopt and adhere to the Mediterranean diet effectively. Remember, it's not just about what you eat but also how you approach meals and your overall lifestyle choices that contribute to its success.

20 HEALTHY SHOPPING INGREDIENTS FOR A MEDITERRANEAN DIET FOR CHRONIC KIDNEY DISEASE PATIENTS

1. **<u>Olive Oil:</u>** A staple in the Mediterranean diet, it's high in heart-healthy fats and antioxidants.

2. **<u>Fish:</u>** Salmon, sardines, and mackerel are excellent sources of omega-3 fatty acids and high-quality protein.

3. **<u>Lean Proteins:</u>** Skinless poultry, eggs, and plant-based proteins like legumes and tofu are good alternatives to red meat.

4. **<u>Whole Grains:</u>** Brown rice, quinoa, bulgur, and whole grain pasta provide fiber and essential nutrients.

5. **Fresh Vegetables:** Bell peppers, spinach, kale, and broccoli are rich in vitamins, minerals, and antioxidants.

6. **Fresh Fruits:** Berries, apples, citrus fruits, and grapes offer vitamins and fiber while being low in potassium.

7. **Herbs and Spices:** Use basil, oregano, rosemary, and turmeric to flavor dishes without adding sodium.

8. **Nuts and Seeds:** Almonds, walnuts, chia seeds, and flaxseeds are healthy sources of fats, fiber, and protein.

9. **Low-Potassium Fruits:** Choose fruits like berries, apples, and grapes that are lower in potassium.

10. **Low-Potassium Vegetables:** Cauliflower, cabbage, and onions are lower in potassium compared to some other veggies.

11. **Low-Sodium Canned Beans:** Rinse them well to reduce sodium content before using in recipes.

12. **Low-Sodium Broths:** Use these as a base for soups and stews instead of high-sodium options.

13. **Low-Fat Dairy or Dairy Alternatives:** opt for low-fat or almond milk, yogurt, or cheese in moderation.

14. **Eggs:** A versatile protein source that's relatively low in potassium and phosphorus.

15. **Whole Wheat Bread:** Choose bread made with whole grains to boost fiber intake.

16. **Garlic:** Adds flavor without extra sodium and offers potential health benefits.

17. **Vinegar:** Use in dressings or marinades for flavor without added salt.

18. **Tea:** Herbal or green teas can be refreshing, and some studies suggest they may have health benefits.

19. **Dark Chocolate:** In moderation, it can satisfy sweet cravings and provide antioxidants.

20. **Water:** Staying hydrated is crucial for kidney health, so drink plenty of water within your doctor's recommended limits.

Always consult with a healthcare professional or a registered dietitian specializing in CKD to tailor these ingredients and portions to your specific dietary needs and restrictions. CKD often requires personalized dietary adjustments based on individual health status and stage of the disease.

CHAPTER THREE

COMPLICATION'S CHRONIC KIDNEY DISEASE, IF THE RIGHT DIET IS NOT ADOPTED

when someone with chronic kidney disease (CKD) doesn't follow an appropriate diet, several complications can arise due to the kidneys' reduced ability to filter waste products and maintain the body's balance of fluids and electrolytes. Here are some potential complications:

1. **Fluid Retention:** When the kidneys can't effectively remove excess fluids, it can lead to swelling in the legs, hands, face, or other parts of the body.

2. **Electrolyte Imbalance:** The kidneys regulate electrolytes like potassium, sodium, and phosphorus. Without proper control, imbalances can occur, leading to muscle cramps, weakness, irregular heartbeat, and even heart problems.

3. **High Blood Pressure:** CKD can cause or worsen high blood pressure. A poor diet can exacerbate this condition, leading to an increased risk of heart disease and stroke.

4. **Bone Health Issues:** When the kidneys are impaired, they can't convert vitamin D into its active form, affecting calcium absorption and leading to weakened bones and an increased risk of fractures.

5. **Anemia:** Healthy kidneys produce a hormone called erythropoietin, which stimulates the production of red blood cells. In CKD, this hormone production decreases, leading to anemia, causing fatigue and weakness.

6. **Uremia:** Buildup of waste products in the blood due to poorly functioning kidneys can lead to symptoms like nausea, vomiting, loss of appetite, and overall feeling unwell.

7. **Cardiovascular Problems:** CKD increases the risk of heart disease. If a proper diet isn't followed, the risk can further elevate due to factors like increased fluid retention, electrolyte imbalances, and high blood pressure.

8. **Malnutrition:** Inadequate intake of essential nutrients due to dietary restrictions or loss of appetite can lead to malnutrition, weakening the body's ability to fight infections and heal.

Adhering to a kidney-friendly diet can help manage these complications by controlling fluid retention, regulating electrolytes, reducing the workload on the kidneys, and managing related health conditions like high blood pressure and diabetes. This diet typically involves controlling intake of protein, sodium, potassium, and phosphorus, while ensuring adequate nutrition to support overall health. It's essential for individuals with CKD to work closely with a registered dietitian or healthcare professional to tailor a diet plan that meets their specific needs based on their stage of CKD, overall health, and other individual factors.

CHAPTER FOUR

BREAKFAST

here are ten Mediterranean-inspired breakfast recipes suitable for individuals with chronic kidney disease. These recipes focus on kidney-friendly ingredients and are relatively easy to prepare:

MEDITERRANEAN VEGGIE OMELET

Number of serving 2   **Cooking Time: 20 minutes**

Ingredients:

1. four eggs
2. One tiny, finely sliced onion
3. One-third cup, one teaspoon of salt
4. 1/8 teaspoon finely powdered black pepper, fresh
5. one finely sliced bell pepper, green
6. two teaspoons of milk

7. Two tablespoons of butter

8. Swiss cheese, shredded, two ounces

Directions:

1. First, prepare by melting one tablespoon of butter in a medium-sized skillet over medium heat.

2. Simmer and mix onion and bell pepper in butter for 4 to 5 minutes, or until they are somewhat soft.

3. After moving the veggies to a bowl and seasoning them with 1/4 teaspoon salt, set them aside.

4. In another bowl, beat eggs, milk, pepper, and the remaining 1/2 teaspoon salt together.

5. Melt the last tablespoon of butter in the skillet over medium heat, swirling to coat the skillet's bottom.

6. Pour the egg mixture into the bubbling butter and heat, stirring occasionally, for one minute or until the bottoms of the eggs start to set.

7. Using a spatula, carefully lift the omelet's edges so that any raw egg spills over onto the skillet.

8. Cook for a further one to two minutes, or until the omelet's center begins to look dry.

9. After spooning the veggie mixture over half of the omelet, sprinkle cheese on top.

10. Fold omelet gently over vegetables with spatula.

11. Simmer for around a minute or until the cheese melts to the right consistency.

12. Omelet is slid onto a plate. Serve after chopping in half.

Nutritional Value

Calories 386g, Fat 30g

Carbs 9g, Protein 22g

GREEK YOGURT PARFAIT

Servings: 8   **Cooking Time: 10 minutes**

Ingredients:

1. 4 cups nonfat plain Greek yogurt

2. 1 cup granular sucralose sweetener (such as Splenda)

3. 1 ½ teaspoons vanilla extract

4. 2 cups granola cereal

5. 8 cups frozen mixed fruit, no sugar added

Direction:

Put the yogurt, sugar, and vanilla extract into a big bowl. Make a good stir.

Fill each of the eight plastic glasses with one cup of frozen fruit. Add a half-cup of the yogurt mixture to each. Keep refrigerated until required.

Before consuming, sprinkle 1/4 cup of granola over each cup of fruit and yogurt.

Nutritional Value:

Calories 359g, Fat 8g

Carbs 61g, Protein 14g

Recipe Tip: you can use any favorite frozen fruit

QUINOA BREAKFAST BOWL

1 serving **Cooking Time: 40 minutes**

Ingredients:

1. 1 cup granular sucralose sweetener (such as Splenda)

2. 1 ½ teaspoons vanilla extract

3. 2 cups granola cereal

4. 8 cups frozen mixed fruit, no sugar added

5. Preparation:

6. Combine yogurt, sweetener, and vanilla extract in a large bowl. Stir well.

7. Place 1 cup of frozen fruit in each of 8 plastic cups. Top each with 1/2 cup yogurt mixture. Store in the refrigerator until needed.

8. Top each cup of fruit and yogurt with 1/4 cup granola before eating.

9. Half a cup of water

10. half a cup of colorful quinoa

11. Half a cup low-sodium cottage cheese

12. One quarter of a banana, cut into slices

13. One spoonful of newly picked blueberries

14. One tsp of chia seeds

15. One pinch of ground cinnamon

Direction:

1. In a saucepan, bring the water and quinoa to a boil.

2. After 15 to 20 minutes, or until the quinoa is soft, reduce heat to medium-low, cover, and simmer.

3. Let cool for a few minutes. In a bowl, mix 1/2 cup of quinoa with cottage cheese. Bananas, blueberries, chia seeds, and cinnamon make great accessories.

4. Combine and proceed to serve.

Nutritional Value:

Calories 313g, Fat 5g

Carbs 48g, Protein 21g

Tip: You can top this with other fruit, 1 to 2 teaspoons low-sugar jam etc

MEDITERRANEAN FRITTATA

Servings: 8   **Cooking Time: 45 minutes**

Ingredients:

1. One 12-oz package of chicken sausage, cut into half-inch rounds
2. ½ cups of zucchini, sliced
3. Half a cup of grape tomatoes

4. Diced red onion, ½ cup
5. One tablespoon of olive oil
6. Twelve big eggs
7. one cup of milk
8. 1/4 tsp kosher salt
9. ½ teaspoon of black pepper, ground
10. ¼ cup of feta cheese in crumbles
11. One tablespoon of freshly chopped dill

Direction:

1. Set the oven's temperature to 400 degrees Fahrenheit (200 degrees Celsius).

2. Arrange the red onion, grape tomatoes, sausage, and zucchini on a baking sheet with a rim.

3. After adding a little olive oil, combine everything.

4. Make a single layer out of it.

5. Roast for about 7 minutes, or until browned all over in the preheated oven.

6. Take the sausage mixture out of the oven and lower the temperature to 375 degrees Fahrenheit (190 degrees Celsius).

7. Mix the eggs, milk, pepper, and salt in a bowl. Evenly cover the sausage mixture with the pour, then top with feta cheese.

8. Go back to the oven and bake for another 17 to 20 minutes, or until the eggs are set.

9. After adding dill, serve.

Nutritional Value:

Calories 239g, Fat 15g

Carbs 7g, Protein 18g

Tip: use roasted garlic chicken sausage with onion and herbs.

AVOCADO TOAST WITH CRUMBLED CRISPY PANCETTA

Serving 1   **Cooking Time: 23 minutes**

Ingredients:

1. One sliced pancetta slice and one egg
2. one prosciutto slice
3. One toasted slice of rye bread, half a chopped ripe avocado, or to taste, salt and ground black pepper

Direction:

1. Put the pancetta in a big skillet and fry it over medium-high heat for about five minutes, turning it occasionally, until it is evenly browned.
2. blot with a paper towel If desired, drizzle some lemon juice over top.

3. Add two to three inches of water to a big saucepan and bring it to a boil.

4. Keep the water simmering gently and lower the heat to medium-low. Crack the egg into a small bowl, hold the bowl slightly over the water's surface, and carefully slip the egg into the simmering water.

5. Cook for 2 to 3 minutes, or until the yolk thickens and the egg white becomes firm.

6. Using a slotted spoon, take the egg from the water and dab off any extra water on a paper towel.

7. Toast should have prosciutto on it.

8. Top with a thick layer of avocado and sprinkle with salt and pepper.

9. Top with the poached egg and add pancetta.

Nutritional Value:

Calories 417g, Fat 29g

Carbs 25g, Protein 17g

FRUIT AND NUT BREAKFAST SALAD

Serving 4   **Preparation Time: 20 minutes**

Ingredients:

1. One kiwi, cut and peeled

2. one cup of grapes

3. Half a cup of blueberries

4. One chopped peeled and chopped orange; seven chopped strawberries

5. one ½ Red Delicious apple (any apple will do)

6. a half-cup of Greek yogurt

7. ½ cup of walnuts, chopped

8. two to three tablespoons of uncooked honey

Direction:

1. Arrange every fruit in a bowl or on a sizable platter.

2. After spooning Greek yogurt over the fruit, top with walnuts.

3. Drizzle the Greek yogurt and berries with honey.

4. Another option is to start with the Greek yogurt on the platter and then arrange the fruit, almonds, and honey on top.

Nutritional Value:

Fiber, vitamins, antioxidants, and healthy fats.

MEDITERRANEAN BREAKFAST WRAP

Serving 1   **Cooking Time: 10 minutes**

Ingredients:

1. Olive Oil Spinach Eggs

2. Sun-dried tomatoes

3. Red onion, feta cheese, and tortilla

Direction:

1. In a skillet with a little oil, wilt the spinach and set it aside.

2. Transfer the egg to the identical skillet.

3. Thaw and stir-fry before adding seasoning.

4. Put the eggs, spinach, and additional toppings on the wrap.

5. To serve, wrap and cut in half.

Nutritional Value:

Protein, fiber, vitamins, and minerals are among the nutrients.

Tips: Heat the tortilla so it is more pliable, Cook the eggs well, Pat any excess oil from the sun-dried tomatoes with some kitchen paper.

CHIA SEED PUDDING

Serving 4 **Total Time: 8 hours 45 mins+ chilling time**

Ingredients:

1. One cup of unsweetened almond milk with vanilla taste
2. One cup fat-free vanilla yogurt
3. Two tsp of sugar only found in maple syrup
4. One-tsp. pure vanilla extract
5. One-fourth cup chia seeds and one-tsp salt
6. One pint of chopped and hulled strawberries
7. Four tsp of pure maple syrup
8. one-half cup toasted almonds

Direction:

1. In a bowl, combine almond milk, yogurt, 2 tablespoons maple syrup, vanilla, and salt; whisk to blend.

2. Add chia seeds; whisk again to incorporate; let soak for 30 minutes.

3. To disperse the seeds that have settled throughout the mixture, stir the chia seed mixture.

4. Refrigerate the bowl for 8 hours or overnight after covering it with plastic wrap.

5. In a bowl, place the strawberries and drizzle with 4 teaspoons maple syrup. Stir to coat.

6. Stir the strawberries with the almonds.

7. Transfer the chia seed mixture into four bowls and place some of the strawberry mixture on top of each.

Nutritional Value:

Calories 243g, Fat 8g

Carbs 38g, Protein 7g

EGG AND SPINACH BREAKFAST MUFFINS WITH TOMATOES

Serving 1   **Cooking Time: 30 minutes**

Ingredients:

1. Milk, eggs, and garlic powder
2. Powdered inion
3. Cheese Caramelized tomatoes

There are two varieties of muffin tins that you can use to steer clear of this sticky situation:

1. Muffin pans without stickiness. Making sure it remains non-stick is crucial in this situation. It's probably not as non-stick as you'd want if your pan has any scratches on it or if you've used it to make dozens of muffins over the years. You can always get a new non-stick muffin pan if this is the case.

2. muffin pan covered in ceramic. Given that it is the most non-stick pan available, this is most likely the best choice. This is

an excellent ceramic muffin pan, if you don't already own one.

Direction:

Nutritional Value:

Protein, vitamins, and antioxidants.

Tip: You can always line your muffin cups with parchment paper if you're still worried that your egg muffins will stick to the pan. Regular paper liners will not work well since the eggs will adhere to them ruthlessly.

MEDITERRANEAN SMOOTHIE BOWL

Serving 1   **Total Time: 5 minutes**

Ingredients:

1. half a cup of Greek yogurt
2. half a banana
3. 1/4 cup of berry mixture
4. One tablespoon of optional honey and two teaspoons of oats

Direction:

1. To prepare, blend together the oats, banana, berries, and yogurt until smooth.

2. Transfer into a bowl and top with honey, if preferred.

Nutritional Value:

Protein, fiber, vitamins, and antioxidants.

These recipes offer a range of nutrients and flavors while being mindful of ingredients suitable for a kidney-friendly diet. Adjust the portion sizes and ingredients based on individual dietary requirements and restrictions.

CHAPTER FIVE

LUNCH

MEDITERRANEAN CHICKEN SALAD

Serving 1   **Cooking Time: 10 minutes**

Ingredients:

1. ½ cup almonds, blanched and slivered

2. Half a cup of mayonnaise

3. One tablespoon of lemon juice

4. ¼ teaspoon of black pepper, ground

5. Two cups of cooked and chopped chicken meat

6. One celery stalk, cut

Direction:

1. Prepare by gathering each ingredient.

2. Put the almonds into a skillet.

3. Over medium-high heat, toast while shaking often.

4. They burn readily, so keep an eye on them.

5. In a medium bowl, combine mayonnaise, lemon juice, and pepper.

6. Combine with celery, toasted almonds, and chicken.

Nutritional Value:

Calories 779g, Fat 63g

Carbs 8g, Protein 44g

MEDITERRANEAN VEGGIE WRAP

Serving 8   **Total Time: 35 minutes**

Ingredients:

1. One mature avocado, chopped, pitted, and peeled

2. One spoonful of mayonnaise

3. Half a teaspoon of salt

4. One-half teaspoon of powdered garlic

5. One-half teaspoon of onion powder

6. 1/2 tsp cayenne pepper, or according to taste

7. Eight eight-inch flour tortillas

8. Two tomatoes, one chopped cucumber, one sliced green bell pepper, and one chopped into strips

9. One chopped head of lettuce and one (8-ounce) container of fresh mozzarella cheese

Direction:

1. To prepare the spread, use a fork to thoroughly mash the diced avocado, mayonnaise, salt, onion powder, garlic powder, and cayenne pepper in a bowl.

2. To assemble the wraps, put a layer of avocado spread on the tortillas.

3. Leaving about 2 inches of room at the bottom of each wrap, top with chopped tomatoes, cucumber slices, bell pepper strips, lettuce, and slices of mozzarella cheese.

4. Turn up the bottoms. Tightly roll tortillas over veggies to enclose fillings.

Nutritional Value:

Fiber, vitamins, and antioxidants.

Tip: Warm tortillas if desired (for flexibility), though it should not be necessary if the wrap is big enough.

TUNA AND WHITE BEAN SALAD

Serving 4   **Total Time: 10 minutes**

Ingredients:

1. Two 6-ounce cans of oil-packed tuna

2. Three cups of washed and drained canned white beans (from two 15-ounce cans), ideally cannellini

3. One thinly chopped red onion

4. 1 tablespoon of capers, drained

5. Two quart-sized bunches of watercress (about 3/4 pound), with the tough stems removed and the greens sliced

6. Two tsp olive oil

7. One tablespoon of vinegar from red or white wine

8. three-quarters teaspoon of salt

9. One tsp freshly ground pepper

Direction:

1. To prepare, combine the beans, onion, capers, watercress, olive oil, vinegar, salt, and pepper in a big bowl together with the tuna and its oil.

2. Gently toss to mix.

Nutritional Value:

Protein, fiber, vitamins, and omega-3 fatty acids.

Tip: If the amount of oil in your tuna can is less than 1.5 tablespoons, top it out with a little extra olive oil. That much oil is what we're depending on for the dressing. You want to use particularly fine canned beans for this salad because there aren't many components and lower-quality beans get mushy. Goya is one of the many excellent brands that we believe to be constantly dependable.

MEDITERRANEAN QUINOA SALAD

Serving 6   **Preparation Time: 35 minutes**

Ingredients:

1. limes and quinoa oil

2. Green onions and cherry tomatoes:

3. Dark beans

4. Adding flavor

Direction:

1. Prepare the quinoa.

2. Prepare the dressing.

3. Add the green onions, black beans, and tomatoes to the quinoa.

4. Mix the other ingredients into the salad after tossing it with the dressing.

Nutritional Value: Protein, fiber, vitamins, and antioxidants.

Tip: If you're not vegan, add even more protein by adding chunks of chicken or turkey.

MEDITERRANEAN BAKED FISH

Serving 1   **Cooking Time: 20 minutes**

Ingredients:

1. Six ounces of white fish fillet, like halibut or cod

2. One tablespoon of olive oil

3. One tsp of dehydrated oregano

4. half a teaspoon of powdered garlic

5. slices of lemon as a garnish

Directions:

1. Set oven temperature to 375°F (190°C) for preparation.

2. Put the fish on a baking sheet, cover with olive oil, and season with garlic powder and oregano.

3. Bake the fish until it's well done.

Nutritional Value: Protein, omega-3 fatty acids, and antioxidants.

EGGPLANT AND TOMATO PASTA

Serving 2   **Cooking Time: 20 minutes**

Ingredients:

1. Three and a half tablespoons of olive oil

2. One medium-sized to large eggplant, roughly 4 cups, chopped and trimmed

3. freshly ground black pepper and kosher salt

4. One medium onion, around one cup, cut coarsely.

5. Two medium garlic cloves, roughly two teaspoons, chopped or shredded using a microplate

6. One tsp of dried red chili powder

7. One 28-oz can of whole, peeled tomatoes

8. One cup of store-bought or homemade low-sodium chicken stock or water

9. three cups of spaghetti penne

10. 1/2 cup finely chopped, packed basil leaves

11. One 4-oz fresh mozzarella ball

Directions:

1. In a 12-inch skillet over medium-high heat, heat 3 tablespoons of oil until shimmering.

2. Add the eggplant and a big teaspoon of salt. Cook, shaking and tossing occasionally, for 10 to 11 minutes, or until the eggplants are fully softened and golden.

3. Simmer the eggplant on medium if it looks like it might burn. Move to a bowl, place foil over it, and leave it there.

4. Turn up the heat to medium-high after adding the last of the oil to the pan.

5. Add a pinch of salt and the onions when they start to shimmer. Cook for about 3 minutes, stirring regularly, or until the onions are tender.

6. After adding the garlic and red chili flakes, simmer for about 30 seconds, or until aromatic.

7. Simmer after adding the tomatoes and their juice.

8. Using a potato masher, carefully break apart the tomatoes once they have softened. Simmer for 8 to 10 minutes, or until

the sauce has thickened and is seasoned to taste. After that, pour in the broth and cook it gently.

9. Make sure there are active, strong bubbles while you add the pasta and cover the pan over medium heat.

10. After cooking the pasta for 12 to 15 minutes, or until it is firm to the bite, stir in the eggplant and stir again to ensure the sauce isn't sticking.

11. Cut the mozzarella into little pieces and place it in the pan. Heat it for about a minute, or until it begins to melt.

12. Add the basil, add salt and pepper to taste, and serve.

Nutritional Value: Fiber, vitamins, and antioxidants.

MEDITERRANEAN LENTIL SOUP

Serving 8   **Cooking Time: 1 hour 35 minutes**

Ingredients:

1. Half a cup of olive oil

2. One chopped onion and two diced carrots

3. two celery stalks, diced

4. two minced garlic cloves

5. One bay leaf

6. One tsp of dehydrated oregano

7. One tsp of dried basil

8. two cups of lentils, dry

9. Eight glasses of water

10. One can (14.5 oz) of crushed tomatoes

11. ½ cup thinly cut and washed spinach

12. Salt and vinegar, to taste, two tablespoons to taste, grind black pepper

Directions:

1. Heat the oil in a big soup pot over medium heat for preparation.

2. Add the onions, carrots, and celery; simmer and stir for 3 to 5 minutes, or until the onion is soft.

3. Cook for two minutes after adding the garlic, bay leaf, oregano, and basil.

4. Add the tomatoes and water, then stir in the lentils. Heat till boiling.

5. Simmer the lentils for at least an hour on low heat, or until they are soft.

6. Add the spinach just before serving, and let it cook until it wilts.

7. Add vinegar, salt, and pepper to taste, and adjust seasoning as necessary.

Nutritional Value:

Calories 349g, Fat 10g

Carbs 48g, Protein 18g

MEDITERRANEAN GRILLED VEGGIE SKEWERS

Serving 8   **Cooking Time:20 minutes**

Ingredients:

1. One raw pineapple, sliced into pieces

2. Slice two medium zucchinis into 1-inch pieces.

3. Two medium yellow squash, sliced into rounds of one inch

4. 1/4 pound of fresh, entire mushrooms

5. One medium red onion, peeled and chopped

6. Twelve cherry tomatoes

7. One medium red bell pepper, diced

8. Eight bamboo skewers, given a 20-minute soak in water

9. Half a cup of olive oil

10. One-and-a-half tsp dried basil and one-tsp dried oregano

11. Half a teaspoon of salt

12. One-half teaspoon of ground black pepper

Directions:

1. Set a grill on medium heat and give the grates a quick oiling.

2. Alternatively, thread bell pepper pieces, mushrooms, onions, pineapple chunks, zucchini slices, yellow squash slices, tomatoes, and bell pepper slices onto skewers.

3. In a bowl, whisk together olive oil, basil, oregano, salt, and black pepper.

4. Drizzle some of the mixture over the veggies.

5. Grill the skewers with the veggies until they are soft, flipping and baste them with the leftover olive oil mixture after ten to fifteen minutes.

Nutritional Value:

Calories 406g, Fat 19g

Carbs 60g, Protein 7g

MEDITERRANEAN CHICKPEA SALAD

Serving 6   **Total Time: 1 hour 15 minutes**

Ingredients:

1. One pint of small cherry tomatoes, cut in half, two 19-ounce cans of rinsed and drained chickpeas (garbanzos), and ½ cup of crumbled goat-milk feta cheese

2. Three teaspoons of basil leaves, finely shredded

3. two tsp honey

4. three big cloves of minced garlic

5. Three teaspoons of vinegar made from red wine

6. Cider vinegar, three tablespoons

7. Three teaspoons of olive oil

8. ½ teaspoon of black pepper, ground

9. 1/2 tsp cayenne pepper 1/2 tsp salt

Directions:

1. In a large mixing bowl, toss together chickpeas, tomatoes, feta cheese, and basil.

2. To prepare the dressing: To make blending simpler, place the honey in a small glass bowl and microwave for 30 seconds.

3. Add the garlic, salt, black pepper, cayenne, olive oil, red wine vinegar, and cider vinegar and stir.

4. Drizzle the chickpea salad with the dressing and toss to coat. Before serving, place plastic wrap over the mixing bowl and chill it for one hour.

Nutritional Value:

Calories 347, Fat 12g

Carbs 51g, Protein 11g

MEDITERRANEAN STUFFED BELL PEPPERS

Serving 4   **Total Time: 1 hour 40 minutes**

Ingredients:

1. Half a cup of water and a cup of raw white rice

2. Four bell peppers, green

3. one-fourth cup olive oil

4. One chopped onion and eight ounces of textured vegetable protein

5. Two tablespoons of freshly chopped parsley

6. Two cups of sauced tomatoes

7. Add the ground black pepper and salt to taste.

8. Four ounces of mozzarella cheese, shredded

Directions:

1. Rice and water should be combined in a small pot and brought to a boil.

2. After the rice is soft and the liquid has been absorbed, reduce the heat to low and simmer for 15 minutes.

3. Raise the oven's temperature to 400°F, or 205°C.

4. Remove the peppers' seeds and cut off the tops. Peppers should be arranged in a big baking dish. Chop off a manageable amount of the tops.

5. The olive oil should be warmed in a large skillet over medium heat.

6. Chopped peppers and onion should be softened in heated oil. Add the parsley and textured vegetable protein and stir. After five minutes, turn down the heat to low and keep cooking. Stir in 1 1/4 cups tomato sauce and cooked rice. Add pepper and salt for seasoning.

7. Fill peppers with mixture; drizzle remaining tomato sauce over each.

8. Bake for approximately 45 minutes with a cover on in a preheated oven.

9. Remove the cover, add mozzarella cheese to the top of each pepper, and bake for an additional five minutes or until the cheese has melted.

Nutritional Value:

Calories 532, Fat 21g

Carbs 38g, Protein 57g.

These lunch recipes offer a variety of flavors and nutrients while aligning with a kidney-friendly diet. Remember to adjust portions and ingredients based on individual dietary requirements and consult with a healthcare professional or dietitian for personalized advice.

CHAPTER SIX

DINNER

Here are ten Mediterranean-inspired dinner recipes suitable for individuals with chronic kidney disease, emphasizing kidney-friendly ingredients and flavors:

MEDITERRANEAN GRILLED CHICKEN

Serving 6   **Cooking Time: 1 hour 30 minutes**

Ingredients:

1. One-third cup of vegetable oil

2. Lime juice, two tablespoons

3. 1/4 tsp finely grated lime zest

4. two smashed garlic cloves

5. 1-1/2 tsp fresh oregano

6. 1/4 teaspoon of flakes red pepper

7. One-tsp salt and one-half tsp ground black pepper

8. Six chicken breast halves, skin and bones removed

Directions:

1. Combine the oil, lime juice, zest, garlic, oregano, red pepper flakes, salt, and black pepper in a shallow glass dish.

2. Turn chicken over to coat. Turning occasionally, marinate in the refrigerator for one hour with a cover on.

3. Set the grill's temperature to medium-high.

4. Give the grill grate a little oil. Remove and dispose of marinade. Until the juices flow clear, grill the chicken for 6 to 8 minutes on each side.

Nutritional Value:

Calories 242, Fat 15g

Carbs 1g, Protein 25g

ROASTED SALMON WITH HERBS

Serving 6   **Cooking Time: 48 minutes**

Ingredients:

1. One skinless (2 to 2 1/2 pound) salmon fillet

2. freshly ground black pepper and kosher salt

3. 1/4 cup of high-quality olive oil

4. two tsp freshly extracted lemon juice

5. Minced green and white sections of 1/2 cup of scallions (4 scallions)

6. ½ cup finely chopped fresh dill

7. ½ cup finely chopped fresh parsley

8. one-fourth cup of dry white wine

9. slices of lemon, for serving

Directions:

1. Set the oven's temperature to 425.

2. Season the salmon fillet with a sufficient amount of salt and pepper and place it on a roasting dish made of glass, ceramic, or stainless steel.

3. Mix the lemon juice and olive oil together, then evenly pour the mixture over the salmon.

4. Give it fifteen minutes to stand at room temperature.

5. Combine the parsley, dill, and scallions in a small basin. Distribute the herb mixture onto the salmon fillet, rotating it so that the green herbs are well coated on all sides.

6. Drizzle the fish fillet with the wine.

7. The thickest section of the salmon should be almost cooked after 10 to 12 minutes of roasting.

8. There will be a line of raw salmon in the very center, but the center will be firm. (I stick the tip of a little knife in to have a peek.) After securing the dish snugly with aluminum foil, give it ten minutes to rest.

9. Slice the salmon crosswise into portions for serving, and then warm it up with lemon wedges.

Nutritional Value:

Calories 449, Total Fat 32g, Saturated Fat 6g

Carbohydrates 2g, Dietary Fiber 1g, Protein 35g

Cholesterol 94mg, Sodium 488mg

MEDITERRANEAN VEGETABLE STIR-FRY

Serving 6   Prep time: 5 minutes   Cooking Time: 5 minutes

Ingredients:

1. Two tsp soy sauce

2. One-third cup brown sugar

3. Two tsp of peanut butter

4. two tsp powdered garlic

5. two tsp olive oil

6. One package (16 ounces) of frozen mixed vegetables

Directions:

1. In a small bowl, mix together soy sauce, brown sugar, peanut butter, and garlic powder.

2. In a big skillet, heat the oil over medium heat. Cook and stir frozen mixed vegetables for 5 to 7 minutes, or until they are just soft.

3. Take off the heat and whisk in the soy sauce blend.

Nutritional Value:

88 Calories, 3g Fat, 14g Carbs, 4g Protein

MEDITERRANEAN QUINOA STUFFED PEPPERS

Servings 6   **Prep Time: 30 mins**

Cook Time: 50 mins   **Total Time:1 hour 20 mins**

Ingredients:

1. One cup of rinsed and drained quinoa

2. two cups of water

3. Two tsp olive oil

4. One little onion, chopped

5. two minced garlic cloves

6. One chopped zucchini

7. One little eggplant, chopped; one tomato, chopped; one cup tomato sauce

8. To taste, add salt and ground black pepper.

9. Six bell peppers, quartered and seeded

10. To taste, use up to 1 cup of shredded mozzarella cheese.

Directions:

1. In a saucepan, combine the quinoa and water; bring to a boil. After the quinoa is soft and the water has been absorbed, cover, lower the heat, and simmer for about 15 minutes.

2. In a large skillet over medium heat, heat the olive oil; sauté and toss the onion and garlic for 5 to 7 minutes, or until aromatic and starting to turn translucent.

3. Cook for 3 to 5 minutes, or until the zucchini, eggplant, and tomato are slightly soft.

4. Mix the tomato sauce with the vegetable mixture, cover, and simmer for an additional 10 minutes or until the veggies are tender.

5. Mix quinoa into the combination of vegetables.

6. Add pepper and salt for seasoning. Pack the quinoa-vegetable mixture into bell peppers.

7. Transfer peppers to baking dish. Wrap the dish in aluminum foil.

8. Bake for about 18 minutes, or until bell peppers are just beginning to soften, in a preheated oven.

9. Take off the aluminum foil cover and add mozzarella cheese to the peppers.

10. Allow the cheese to melt and bubble for a further five minutes in the oven.

Nutritional Value:

Calories 251g, Fat 10g

Carbs 32g, Protein 11g

LEMON GARLIC SHRIMP PASTA

Servings: 6   **Prep Time: 10 mins**

Cook Time: 15 mins   **Total Time: 2 hours 25 mins**

Ingredients:

1. Half a cup of kosher salt
2. One gallon of cold water

3. Two pounds of big shrimp, peeled and deveined (between 21 and 30 per pound)

4. One package (16 ounces) of angel hair pasta

5. One-half cup unsalted butter

6. Half a cup of olive oil

7. three teaspoons of finely chopped garlic

8. One-third cup white wine

9. Half a cup of lemon juice

10. A tsp of finely ground red pepper flakes

11. One teaspoon of finely powdered black pepper

12. ½ cup of freshly chopped parsley

13. One tablespoon of zest from lemons

Directions:

1. In a large pot, dissolve the kosher salt in one gallon of water.

2. After adding the shrimp, chill for two to four hours. Shake well and use paper towels to pat shrimp dry.

3. Lightly salted water should be added to a big saucepan and heated to a rolling boil over high heat.

4. After bringing the water to a boil, add the angel hair pasta and bring it back to a boil.

5. Cook the pasta, uncovered, stirring now and again, for 4 to 5 minutes, or until it is cooked through but still has some bite to it. In a colander placed in the sink, thoroughly drain.

6. In the meantime, heat a large skillet over medium-low heat and melt the butter and olive oil.

7. Add the garlic and simmer for 3 to 4 minutes, or until it becomes soft. Stir in the red pepper flakes, lemon juice, white wine, and shrimp.

8. Simmer and stir for approximately 6 minutes, or until the shrimp becomes opaque in the middle.

9. Toss with the angel hair pasta and stir in the lemon zest, parsley, and black pepper.

Nutritional Value:

Total Fat 20g, Saturated Fat 7g

Cholesterol 251mg, Sodium 11829mg

Total Carbohydrate 45g, Dietary Fiber 3g

Total Sugars 2g, Protein 33g, Vitamin C 17mg

Calcium 87mg, Iron 6mg, Potassium 449mg

MEDITERRANEAN BAKED EGGPLANT

Servings: 6   **Prep Time: 15 mins**

Cook Time: 35 mins   **Total Time: 50 mins**

Ingredients:

1. cooking oil

2. One eggplant, cut into rounds that are 1/2 inch thick.

3. Three sliced tomatoes

4. One tablespoon of pure olive oil

5. One teaspoon each of ground black pepper and oregano salt, to taste

6. Grated Parmesan cheese, ⅓ cup

Directions:

1. Set the oven's temperature to 400°F, or 200°C. Grease a baking dish with nonstick cooking spray.

2. Place the tomato and eggplant slices in the bottom of the baking dish that has been prepared. Add a drizzle of olive oil and season the vegetables with salt, pepper, and oregano. Add a sprinkling of Parmesan cheese.

3. Bake for about 30 minutes in a preheated oven, or until the cheese starts to brown.

4. Turn the oven broiler up to high and keep baking for about five minutes, or until the top is nicely browned.

Nutritional Value:

Total Fat 4g, Saturated Fat 1g

Cholesterol 4mg, Sodium 72mg

Total Carbohydrate 3g, Dietary Fiber 1g

Total Sugars 2g, Protein 2g

Vitamin C 10mg, Calcium 61mg

Iron 0mg, Potassium 185mg

MEDITERRANEAN BEAN SOUP

Servings: 8   **Prep Time: 25 mins**

Cook Time: 1 hour 40 mins   **Total Time: 2 hours 5 mins**

Ingredients:

1. One bag (16 ounces) of dry navy beans

2. Seven glasses of water

3. One bone of ham

4. 1/2 cup minced onion and 2 cups chopped ham

5. A tsp of salt and a sprinkle of black pepper

6. One bay leaf

7. ½ cup of carrots, sliced

8. Half a cup of sliced celery

Directions:

1. To prepare, rinse the beans, then move them to a large stockpot and pour in water.

2. After 2 minutes of simmering and bringing to a boil, turn off the heat, cover, and leave for 1 hour.

3. Add the onion, cubed ham, bay leaf, salt, and pepper. Bring to a boil, then lower the heat to a simmer, cover, and cook for one hour and fifteen minutes, or until the beans are tender.

4. Cook the celery and carrots for ten to fifteen minutes, or until they are soft.

5. When the ham bone is cold enough to handle, remove it from the saucepan and lay it on a chopping board.

6. Cut any flesh off the bones into bite-sized pieces, then stir the meat back into the soup to reheat it.

Nutritional Value:

Daily Value

Calories 247

Total Fat 4g, Saturated Fat 1g

Cholesterol 17mg, Sodium 543mg

Total Carbohydrate 37g, Dietary Fiber 14g

Total Sugars 3g, Protein 17g

Vitamin C 3mg, Calcium 98mg

Iron 3mg, Potassium 809mg

MEDITERRANEAN RATATOUILLE

Servings: 4 **Prep Time: 15 mins**

Cook Time: 45 mins **Total Time: 1 hour**

Ingredients:

1. 2 tbsp olive oil, split into 3 cloves of garlic, minced, and chopped into 1/2-inch cubes of eggplant

2. Two tsp salt-dried parsley, according to taste

3. Grated Parmesan cheese, one cup

4. Two sliced zucchinis

5. two big tomatoes, cut up

6. Two cups of freshly sliced mushrooms

7. One big onion cut into rings

8. 1 sliced bell pepper, either red or green

Directions:

1. Set the oven to 175 degrees Celsius, or 350 degrees Fahrenheit.

2. Grease a 1-1/2-quart casserole dish from bottom to side with one tablespoon of olive oil.

3. In a medium skillet, heat the remaining tablespoon of olive oil over medium heat.

4. Garlic is cooked and stirred until aromatic and golden brown.

5. After adding the eggplant and parsley, heat and stir for ten minutes or until the eggplant is soft and tender. Add salt to taste to season.

6. Evenly distribute the eggplant mixture in the bottom of the casserole dish that has been prepared, then top with a few tablespoons of Parmesan cheese.

7. Evenly distribute the zucchini on top. Season with a little salt and add a bit extra cheese.

8. Continue layering in this manner with the bell pepper, onion, mushrooms, and tomatoes, finishing each layer with a sprinkle of cheese and salt.

9. Bake for 45 minutes or until vegetables are soft in a preheated oven.

Nutritional Value:

Daily Value

Calories 251, Saturated Fat 5g

Total Fat 14g, Cholesterol 18mg

Sodium 327mg, Total Carbohydrate 24g

Dietary Fiber 7g, Total Sugars 13g

Protein 13g, Vitamin C 56mg

Calcium 271mg, Iron 2mg

Potassium 1049mg

GREEK LEMON CHICKEN SKEWERS

Servings: 4

Prep Time: 20 mins

Cook Time: 20 mins

Total Time: 2 hours 40 mins

1.Ingredients:

2. 1/4 cup of lemon juice

3. 1/4 cup of wok oil

4. A ⅛ cup of red wine vinegar

5. One tablespoon of onion powder

6. One tablespoon of finely chopped garlic

7. One freshly squeezed lemon

8. one tsp of Greek seasoning

9. one tsp poultry seasoning

10. One tsp. of dried oregano

11. One tsp finely ground black pepper

12. 1/2 tsp. dried thyme

13. Three skinless, boneless chicken breasts, or chop into 1-inch pieces as needed

14. Eight bamboo skewers, soaked in water for half an hour, or more if necessary

Directions:

1. Lemon juice, oil, vinegar, garlic, onion flakes, lemon zest, Greek seasoning, poultry seasoning, oregano, pepper, and thyme should all be combined in a bowl before being poured into a plastic bag that can be sealed.

2. Squeeze out extra air from the chicken, add it, cover with marinade, and close the bag. For a minimum of two hours, marinate in the fridge.

3. Turn the oven's temperature up to 350 degrees Fahrenheit (175°C).

4. Take the chicken out of the marinade, shake off any excess, and then thread it onto skewers. Throw away any marinade that remains. Place the skewers on a baking sheet.

5. Roast for approximately 20 minutes in a preheated oven, or until golden brown.

Note: You can alternatively roast the skewers over a grill. Lightly oil the grates of an outdoor grill and preheat it to medium heat. As the grill preheats, cook the skewers, rotating them from time to time, until the internal temperature of an instant-read thermometer reaches 165 degrees Fahrenheit (74 degrees Celsius).

Nutritional Value:

Daily Value

Calories 248 Total Fat 17g

Saturated Fat 3g, Cholesterol 49mg

Sodium 167mg, Total Carbohydrate 4g

Dietary Fiber 1g, Total Sugars 1g

Protein 18g, Vitamin C 9mg

Calcium 29mg, Iron 1mg, Potassium 215mg

MEDITERRANEAN BAKED COD

Servings: 4 **Prep Time: 10 mins**

Cook Time: 25 mins **Total Time: 35 mins**

Ingredients:

1. 4 tablespoons butter, divided; crush 1 pound of thickly sliced cod loin; and ½ sleeve buttery round crackers.

2. ½ cup dry white wine; ½ medium lemon, juiced

3. 1 tablespoon of freshly chopped parsley

4. One tablespoon of finely sliced green onions

5. One medium lemon, thinly sliced

Directions:

1. assemble all components for preparation.

2. Preheat the oven to 400 degrees Celsius, or Fahrenheit.

3. Put two tablespoons of butter in a bowl that can be microwaved. To melt in 30 seconds or less on high in the microwave. Mix melted butter with buttery round crackers.

4. In a 7 by 11-inch baking dish, add the final 2 tablespoons of butter. In a preheated oven, melt for one to three minutes. Take out the dish from the oven.

5. Coat the cod in the baking dish with melted butter on both sides.

6. For ten minutes, bake the cod in the preheated oven.

7. Pull the food out of the oven. sprinkle the wine, lemon juice, and cracker mixture on top. Put the fish back in the oven and bake for a further 10 minutes or until it becomes opaque and flakes easily with a fork.

8. Add some parsley and green onion as garnish, and serve with lemon wedges.

Nutritional Value:

Daily Value

Calories 280, Total Fat 16g

Saturated Fat 8g, Cholesterol 72mg

Sodium 282mg, Total Carbohydrate 9g

Total Sugars 1g, Protein 21g

Vitamin C 7mg, Calcium 25mg

Iron 1mg, Potassium 410mg

These dinner recipes offer a variety of flavors and nutrients while aligning with a kidney-friendly diet. Adjust portions and ingredients based on individual dietary requirements and consult with a healthcare professional or dietitian for personalized advice.

SNACKS

MEDITERRANEAN CUCUMBER AND YOGURT DIP

Ingredients:

1 cup Greek yogurt

1/2 cucumber (peeled and diced)

1 tablespoon chopped dill

1 clove garlic (minced)

Preparation:

Mix yogurt, cucumber, dill, and garlic in a bowl.

Serve chilled with vegetable sticks.

Nutritional Value: Protein, probiotics, vitamins, and antioxidants.

Time: 10 minutes

HUMMUS AND VEGGIE STICKS

Ingredients:

1 cup hummus

Carrot sticks, cucumber slices, bell pepper strips

Preparation:

Serve hummus with assorted vegetable sticks for dipping.

Nutritional Value: Fiber, protein, vitamins, and antioxidants.

Time: 5 minutes

GREEK SALAD SKEWERS

Ingredients:

Cherry tomatoes

Cucumber chunks

Feta cheese cubes

Kalamata olives (pitted)

Preparation:

Thread cherry tomatoes, cucumber, feta, and olives onto skewers.

Nutritional Value: Vitamins, calcium, antioxidants, and healthy fats.

Total Time: 10 minutes

MEDITERRANEAN EDAMAME

Ingredients:

1 cup cooked edamame

1 tablespoon olive oil

Salt and pepper (to taste)

Preparation:

Toss cooked edamame with olive oil, salt, and pepper.

Nutritional Value: Protein, fiber, vitamins, and healthy fats.

Preparation Time: 5 minutes

YOGURT AND BERRY PARFAIT

Ingredients:

1 cup Greek yogurt

1/4 cup mixed berries

1 tablespoon chopped nuts (almonds or walnuts)

1 teaspoon honey (optional)

Preparation:

Layer yogurt, berries, and nuts in a glass.

Drizzle honey on top if desired.

Nutritional Value: Protein, calcium, antioxidants, and healthy fats.

Time: 5 minutes

DESSERTS

MEDITERRANEAN FRUIT SALAD

Ingredients:

1 cup mixed fruits (berries, apples, grapes)

1 tablespoon chopped mint

1 tablespoon honey (optional)

Preparation:

Mix fruits and mint in a bowl.

Drizzle honey on top if desired.

Nutritional Value: Vitamins, antioxidants, and natural sweetness.

Time: 5 minutes

GREEK YOGURT POPSICLES

Ingredients:

1 cup Greek yogurt

1/4 cup mixed berries (blended)

1 tablespoon honey (optional)

Preparation:

Mix yogurt, blended berries, and honey in a bowl.

Pour into popsicle molds and freeze until set.

Nutritional Value: Protein, calcium, antioxidants, and natural sweetness.

Time: 10 minutes + freezing time

ALMOND AND DATE ENERGY BALLS

Ingredients:

1 cup almonds (blanched)

1 cup dates (pitted)

1 tablespoon unsweetened cocoa powder

Preparation:

Blend almonds, dates, and cocoa powder in a food processor until a dough forms.

Roll into small balls and refrigerate.

Nutritional Value: Fiber, protein, vitamins, and natural sweetness.

Time: 15 minutes

MEDITERRANEAN ORANGE SLICES WITH CINNAMON

Ingredients:

Orange slices

Ground cinnamon

Preparation:

Sprinkle orange slices with ground cinnamon.

Nutritional Value: Vitamins, antioxidants, and natural sweetness.

Time: 5 minutes

BAKED APPLES WITH CINNAMON

Ingredients:

2 apples (cored and sliced)

1 teaspoon cinnamon

1 tablespoon honey (optional)

Preparation:

Place apple slices in a baking dish, sprinkle with cinnamon.

Drizzle with honey if desired, bake until tender.

Nutritional Value: Vitamins, antioxidants, and natural sweetness.

Time: 20 minutes

These snack and dessert recipes offer a balance of nutrients and flavors while being mindful of ingredients suitable for a kidney-friendly diet. Adjust portions and ingredients based on individual dietary requirements and consult with a healthcare professional or dietitian for personalized advice.

CONCLUSION

In the world of managing chronic kidney disease (CKD), the Mediterranean diet stands as a beacon of hope and healing. This cookbook harnesses the essence of Mediterranean cuisine, offering an array of delectable recipes tailored especially for people navigating the challenges of CKD.

Throughout these pages, you'll find a symphony of flavors meticulously crafted to align with the unique dietary requirements of CKD. From nutrient-rich salads and protein-packed mains to tantalizing snacks and guilt-free sweets, each recipe is a testament to the harmonious fusion of taste and health.

The Mediterranean diet, rooted in whole grains, fresh fruits, vegetables, lean proteins, and healthy fats like olive oil, naturally embodies the principles conducive to kidney health. These recipes favor low sodium, controlled phosphorus and potassium, while maximizing essential nutrients crucial for managing CKD.

Moreover, beyond its nutritional prowess, the Mediterranean diet for CKD offers a route to a more vibrant lifestyle. It's not merely a culinary trip but a holistic approach to wellness. By embracing this dietary shift, you're not just nurturing your body but improving overall well-being. The diet's focus on wholesome, unprocessed ingredients empowers you to take charge of your health, fostering a sense of empowerment and control in the face of a challenging diagnosis.

So, dear reader, within these recipes lies a guide to a healthier tomorrow. By embracing the Mediterranean diet for CKD, you aren't just savoring flavorful meals; you're taking a step towards controlling your condition more effectively. It's an invitation to discover a world where health and taste converge, where each meal becomes a celebration of life and vitality.

Remember, the journey to better health is a set of small steps. Embrace these recipes, enjoy the flavors, and witness the transformative power of nourishing your body and soul with the Mediterranean diet for chronic kidney disease. Let each dish be a reminder of your resolve to a healthier, happier you. Your journey to wellness starts here, with each flavorful creation inviting you to embrace a life of vitality and well-being.

DRY WEIGHTS

			KG
1/2 oz	1 tbsp	-	15 g
1 oz	2 tbsp	1/8 c	28 g
2 oz	4 tbsp	1/4 c	57 g
3 oz	6 tbsp	1/3 c	85 g
4 oz	8 tbsp	1/2 c	115 g
8 oz	16 tbsp	1 cup	227 g
12 oz	24 tbsp	1½ c	340 g
16 oz	32 tbsp	2 c	455 g

1 OZ = 28 GRAMS
1 LBS = 454 G
1 CUP = 227 G

1 TSP = 5 ML
1 TBSP = 15 ML
1 OZ = 30 ML
1 CUP = 237 ML
1 PINT = 473 ML (2 CUPS)
1 GALLON = 16 CUPS

LIQUID VOLUMES

1 oz	2 tbsp	1/8 c	30 ml
2 oz	4 tbsp	1/4 c	60 ml
2⅔ oz	6 tbsp	1/3 c	80 ml
4 oz	8 tbsp	1/2 c	120 ml
8 oz	16 tbsp	2/3 c	160 ml
12 oz	24 tbsp	3/4 c	177 ml
16 oz	32 tbsp	1 cup	237 ml
32 oz	64 tbsp	1½ c	470 ml
		2 c	950 ml

ABBREVIATIONS

tbsp = Tablespoon
tsp = Teaspoon
fl.oz = Fluid Ounce
c = cup
ml = Milliliter
lb = pound
F = Fahrenheit
C = Celsius
ml = Milliliter
g = grams
kg = kilogram
l = liter

BAKING PAN

9-inch (by 3") standard round pan = 12 cups
9-inch (by 2.5") springform pan = 10 cups
10-inch (by 4") tube pan = 16 cups
9-inch (by 3") bundt pan = 12 cups
9-inch (by 2") square pan = 10 cups
9 x 5 inch loaf pan = 8 cups

OVEN TEMP.

130 c = 250 F
165 c = 325 F
177 c = 350 F
190 c = 375 F
200 c = 400 F
220 c = 425 F

Gain access to my other exciting books on this QR CODE, Just scan it as simple as that.

Here is my email QR CODE

Feel free to send me email at

rmillerdorothy51@gmail.com

" If you have any question regarding this book, I will be at your service any day anytime, feedback within two hours."

Please if you can I do really appreciate if you leave me a review if you have the chance after enjoying this book, thank you

www.ingramcontent.com/pod-product-compliance
Lightning Source LLC
Chambersburg PA
CBHW082217290526

45794CB00009B/3569